A U. S. Marine's Manual for

Perfect Weight

The World's Simplest Weight Control System, NOT A Diet

LtCol. Kevin G. Emery, USMC (Ret.)

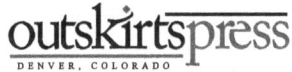

outskirtspress

DENVER, COLORADO

Outskirts Press, Inc.
http://www.outskirtspress.com

ISBN: 978-1-4787-6600-1

Library of Congress Control Number: 2015916524

Outskirts Press and the "OP" logo are trademarks belonging to Outskirts Press, Inc.

PRINTED IN THE UNITED STATES OF AMERICA

Contents

CHAPTER One

Introduction

ALOHA, I AM Lt. Col. Kevin G. Emery, USMC (Ret.), and can tell you from personal experience that this system will work for anyone who follows its simple rules. It is so simple, but very hard to do because you have to change the way you think. Most of you will first scoff at my system and think I am crazy. But it does work and will always work if you honestly and constantly do the simple, easy tasks every day. I challenge anyone to prove to me it does not work if you faithfully do the simple suggestions each day, and believe they will work.

Most diets restrict what and how much you can drink/eat and how often, but this book will NOT tell you any of these restrictions, and most of the time, once you reach your diet goal a month later, you are back to your old weight. Are you now interested in learning about my manual for reaching and maintaining your perfect weight? If you will read this simple book and follow the directions, there is no possible way you will fail. But you must do the same easy things each day, and I mean *every* day, for it to work. This weight loss system requires no calorie counting, tonics, fasting, flushing, starving, wraps, spas, special training, exercise, or anything else the usual diet books preach. Some diets work, but once you lose the weight, it comes back because you have not changed your true picture of yourself. This book will get your mind right so you can maintain your weight loss and keep your perfect weight.

One of my biggest challenges while I was active duty was keeping my weight under the United States Marine Corps (USMC) standards. I could run a first-class Physical Fitness Test (PFT) any day of the week, but the scales were a different story. The mandatory PFT and weigh in was done every six months. So twice each year, I would starve myself for two weeks prior to the PFT, then sit in a sauna until I made the weight. Not to mention I would work out for an hour in the morning (0530–0630) and be at work by 0700. For breakfast, I would eat one orange to keep me going. Then at lunchtime, I would work out again from 1100–1300, then have a salad for lunch and eat little to nothing for dinner. I did this for the last 15 years of my career. Even when I was not getting ready for the PFT, I would work out twice a day. I just would not starve myself, but I always seemed to be five to 15 pounds over my max USMC weight.

When I retired from the Marine Corps, I still kept up my training so I would not gain too much weight. Then, I got a job in the civilian world and exercise was not required. I slowly, over several years, began to put on unwanted weight. I went from my active duty USMC weight of 193–210 pounds to a whopping 275-plus pounds over nine years, and my health was failing. That is when I said to myself, *enough is enough. I must get my act together and lose weight and get back to my USMC active duty weight.* The U.S. Marine in me told me I must win!

I started to read self-help and diet books; additionally, I began to exercise an hour each day, but the weight still just would not come off. Then in my research, I discovered the secret system. I am going to now pass this secret simple system to you, and it will work as sure as the sun comes up each morning. I went from a sickly overweight man of 275-plus pounds back to my perfect weight of 190–200 pounds in a matter of 18 months or less. By the way, 18 months will work for everyone, but some of you may even reach your goal sooner. I am healthy and fit and wrote this book to help others live happier and healthier lives.

Now, are you ready to get started? This should only take you less than 30 minutes to read, so don't be afraid. Like Frank Sinatra said, "Massive Success is the best revenge." Why not show them all, YOU CAN DO IT!

There are two main reasons why I kept this book short. First, I wanted it short enough that you can reread this book each and every day. I want you to highlight or underline the parts that jump out at you so you should be able to reread it very quickly. Second, it will help you start your success journal which is included in the last chapter.

I welcome future testimonials but have not included any but my own. I want to test the student and let you see for yourself this system works. Personal improvement will be far more powerful than anyone else's stories. I will create a follow-on book documenting my future students' successes, and maybe *you* will be one of my successful subjects, with your permission, of course! If you follow the steps and believe, you will be successful in reaching your perfect weight as sure as rain and the sun make rainbows.

This is a practical manual and journal, not a philosophy, religious, or science book. If you want to know all the philosophical theory and quantum physics that are behind my practical lessons, there are thousands of books you can read. This book is based completely on the teachings in the Bible. This book is intended for the women or men whose pressing need is to become their perfect weight and keep it there—so you can feel healthy and happy and live a wonderful life. Let's begin now on your next 18 months (547 days), or less, journey into discovery and success.

Say you want to get to your perfect weight of 135 pounds, but you are currently 225 pounds. That means you only have to lose 90 pounds (1,440 ounces), or just 2.6 ounces per day. I will not reference weight loss again. It all boils down to being a little successful every day in reaching your goal. Then it is mathematically impossible for you to fail.

CHAPTER TWO

Forgiveness

WAKE UP! FORGIVE yourself for being FAT, OVERWEIGHT, ETC. If you cannot forgive yourself, NO ONE can save you! You must also forgive anyone who you might possibly blame for your overweight condition, and that includes age, economy, weather, community, race, Mom, Dad, family, friends, and colleagues . . . you name it. You must take full responsibility for your life and your weight. I do not care if you are a teen or 70-plus years old. If you decide, you can do it. Blame no one else; you make your own life and destiny. The fact that you can believe and accept that you are FAT is 99 percent of the solution.

Now, forget all feelings of being overweight. You have to forgive yourself to move forward and accomplish the mission. If you are constantly beating yourself up about being overweight, what are you thinking about? Yes, *your excess weight*. Make peace with your past mistakes and blaming of others. We become what we think about, so you will never lose the weight because you constantly are thinking negatively about your weight, and you will never break free of this cycle of defeat. That is why diets do not work in the long run. Diets tell you what you can and cannot have, which keeps you in the terrible no-win cycle of being overweight.

The main idea is you must constantly think and believe that you are at your ideal perfect weight . . . NOW. I use the mantra that goes like this: "I AM so Happy and Grateful now that I AM a <u>190 pound</u> healthy, loving, spiritual human being, and I AM getting better and better every day in every way."

Before we set our perfect weight goal, we need to discuss the believable aspect of this weight control system. If, in your heart of hearts, you do not believe you can reach your perfect weight, you never will. You need to pick a weight that is realistic for your age, height, and body type, and most importantly, that you truly believe you can become.

NOW, let us set our goal weight: 135 pounds, for example, for a female. It could be 200 pounds if you are a man. You must decide the weight you want to be, no one else. You want to concentrate your efforts and thinking ONLY on your final desired weight, or your end game, if you will. You must visualize yourself in the end state of your perfect weight (act as if it already is). It must be a believable weight goal for your height and body shape. Remember, this is an 18-month goal, or less. If you have been that weight in the past, it will be easy to believe, but if you were always overweight your whole life, it will be more of a challenge, but I know you can do it because this system never fails if followed.

If YOU DECIDE to change, you will. I believe the hardest thing is to stop having negative thoughts about your weight or anything in your life. Remember the law of attraction which says, "You attract what you think about," so if you have negative thoughts about weight, all you really do is attract the weight of excess food. On the other hand, if you always see yourself in your mind as being at your perfect weight, you will become what you think about all day long . . . (act as if it already is).

Remember to forgive yourself for setbacks, but immediately get back on track of your perfect weight plan.

Everyone knows the Golden Rule very well: "Do unto others that which you would have them do unto you." What does that mean for my manual for perfect weight? It means to always hear and accept as true of others that which you would desire for yourself. In the context of reaching your perfect weight, you should only say and have positive comments and thoughts about others' weight and congratulate improvements you see in others . . .

Bottom line: DO NOT GOSSIP about people in a negative fashion; only think and say loving and positive things about the people you meet and know. Stay away from negative people and hang out with people who are positive and supportive. If you catch yourself talking bad about someone and stop, that is a major breakthrough on you getting the manual's system for perfect weight. Once you catch yourself, say to yourself, "I AM the captain of my thoughts and the master of my body."

CHAPTER Three

Imagination/Visualization

SO, FIRST, YOU must determine what your own personal ideal weight should be. I mean, your final goal weight, not step-by-step nonsense. Pick a weight that you REALLY want and BELIEVE you can reach. Examples: 1. I want to be the weight I was in college or high school, and you then must visualize yourself at that weight. Use your five senses in your vision of yourself at your perfect weight. See the school and your friends; smell the grass; taste the drink; feel the excitement; and hear the other students chatting in your vision. Make it as real as possible for the best results. 2. In your head, visualize yourself in your swimsuit at the pool or beach and see yourself and feel yourself in those conditions at your perfect weight now. Use your five senses in your vision of yourself at your perfect weight. See the pool; smell the water; taste the chlorine; feel the water; and hear the splashing water in your vision. Make it as real as possible for the best results. It is even better if you have a photo of yourself when you were at that weight. 3. Ladies, how about seeing yourself in your wedding dress at your perfect weight? Use your five senses in your vision of yourself at your perfect weight. See the wedding; smell the flowers; taste the cake; feel the silky dress; and hear the music in your vision.

I picked my personal goal weight of 190 pounds, which was my low average, active U.S. Marine Corps weight for 24 years. I used my old photo at that weight to help me visualize myself. I really wanted it and knew I could do it, and I believed I could reach it. I did it—and so CAN YOU!

Remember, the weight must be realistic for you. You will need to take your age, body shape, lifestyle, and desire in setting your perfect weight. This is extremely important because if you cannot truly believe in your gut that you can make your goal perfect weight, you never will. So pick a healthy weight for you as your perfect weight. I picked 190 pounds, like I said before. It is a healthy weight for me, where I am lean but not skinny and ripped, just healthy.

Now, equally important as picking your perfect weight is you MUST be able to imagine yourself looking as if you are your perfect weight in your mind now. This is a MUST; you must see yourself at your perfect weight doing some activity you enjoy, as if you are doing that activity now. Your imagination is one of the keys to success in reaching and maintaining your perfect weight. Use your five senses (sight, sound, touch, smell, and taste) in your vision. That is another reason this system will work, because you are the one driving the train for your success, not someone demanding or telling you to reach your goal.

Before sleeping and upon waking, use your imagination and see yourself enjoying life at your perfect weight goal. It could be bowling, golfing, fishing, or any other activity you enjoy. Imagine your friends telling you how great you look. Be in your own created moment and visualize your success now, even before it happens in reality . . . The more you imagine your success, the better the system works. Just know you are there.

CHAPTER Four

Action

THE LAW OF attraction is another hinge pin to this secret perfect weight system. The last part of the word "attraction" is made up of the word "action," this chapter's namesake. You must take action by following the simple rules in this book for this system to work.

Notice I did not use the words "weight loss system." Why? Because loss is a negative statement or thought. I want you to constantly think of yourself at your perfect weight. You must choose positive and loving thoughts. Life is a constant choice, and you must choose to only give off positive thoughts. Anytime you are hungry or craving some food or candy, say the following: "I AM so Happy and Grateful now that I AM a <u>135 pound</u> healthy, loving, spiritual human being, and I AM getting better and better every day in every way." You need to memorize this statement and say it to yourself constantly (300-plus times each day), especially before you sleep or before taking a nap and always upon awakening. I assure you, your sleep will improve as a side benefit if you repeat the above statement to yourself as you fall asleep. It works a hundred times better than counting sheep or thinking about negative things that happened during the day.

Forget all that junk and repeat "I AM so Happy and Grateful now that I AM a <u>135 pound</u> healthy, loving, spiritual being, and I AM getting better and better every day in every way." Just change the 135 pounds to your own personal perfect weight number. This program is a choice, and once you decide to reach your goal, nothing can stop you . . . Forget setbacks and keep going. Never quit and you will succeed. Never give up!

Guess what will start to happen if you do the above steps? You will naturally, slowly, start doing things in a right way. What do I mean by that? Well, you will decide to begin to eat less without anyone telling you to . . . You will also find yourself compelled to start exercising in small ways you have never done before. These small steps will come naturally to you without your being told or directed to perform them. Why? Because YOU have decided on your perfect weight, and you cannot help but obtain the weight you see yourself to be. You must see yourself at your perfect weight. Look at your goal photo several times each day and always before sleeping and upon awakening.

You may ask, why before I sleep and upon awakening? Well, I will tell you. First, when you sleep, your subconscious mind takes over from your awake mind. When you fall into slumber thinking of good positive pictures of yourself at your perfect weight, your subconscious mind takes it for action and directs your subconscious actions to make your perfect weight happen in a natural way. Be sure to use your five senses of sight, sound, touch, smell, and taste in your vision of your perfect weight. The cool thing about this is you are not constantly stressed out about what you eat. You will naturally cut back, and you will not even be aware of it most, if not all, the time. You will start exercising on your own initiative instead of being told to do it, because you have DECIDED to be your perfect weight. Once you reach your perfect weight, you will maintain your perfect weight because you decided to do it.

Now, why especially in the morning do I want you to repeat: "I AM so Happy and Grateful now that I AM a <u>135 pound</u> healthy, loving, spiritual human being, and I AM getting better and better every day in every way"? Because it gets your day started in a positive way, and it will remind you to repeat "I AM so Happy and Grateful now that I AM a <u>135 pound</u> healthy, loving, spiritual human being, and I AM getting better and better every day in every way" over and over again in your mind, especially when you see or hear anything negative about food. Whenever you catch yourself thinking in a negative way, say the following to yourself: "I AM the captain of my own thoughts and the master of my body," then repeat, numerous times, until your negative thoughts fall away into oblivion. "I AM so Happy and Grateful now that I AM a <u>135 pound</u> healthy, loving, spiritual human being, and I AM getting better and better every day in every way." To many people this sounds crazy—but it works. Now, I will give a word of caution about this whole process. Keep it to yourself. Only tell individuals that support you 100 percent. It is sad, but many people, friends, and even loved ones will not want you to succeed and constantly say negative things about your plan. Leave them out of your perfect weight system.

This brings me to another valuable action step that will improve your progress to your perfect weight. See these naysayers in your dozing just before you sleep congratulating you at how great you look. Imagine your best friend saying to you, "WOW, you look great!" And you say back to them, "Thank you! I AM at my perfect weight of 135 pounds" before and after you repeat to yourself, "I AM so Happy and Grateful that I AM a <u>135 pound</u> healthy, loving, spiritual human being, and I AM getting better and better every day in every way" as you fade into blissful sleep . . .

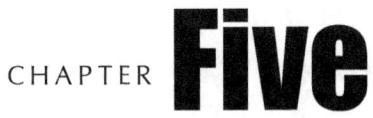

Write It Down

NOW, I WILL cover the final step . . . putting your perfect weight statement down in writing. "So as it is written, so let it be done" is a statement that is very powerful. I want you to write in the space below in your own handwriting the following statement: "I AM so Happy and Grateful now that I AM a _____ pound healthy, loving, spiritual human being, and I AM getting better and better every day in every way." You fill in the blank for your own personal weight. If you can write this on your goal photo, you can have it altogether and look at it multiple times each day, but especially before sleeping and upon awaking.

Also, write down: "I AM the captain of my own thoughts and the master of my body." Read this whenever negative thoughts pop into your mind or someone talks negatively about your goal or perfect weight.

I also want you to write down today's date and the date 18 months from now in your journal. This is when you will be writing me a letter or e-mail telling me about your success story. As a matter of fact, write me your success story, as if it is already done, the first day you begin this system, and read it every day. In 18 months, you can send me the letter or e-mail verifying this information. I am excitedly waiting to hear your results that you decided to create. I look forward to reading and sharing your success. Remember, every morning is the first day of the rest of your life, so never give up! If you make small improvements daily, it is mathematically impossible for you to fail. So keep going, even when you have a setback; keep pushing forward. That is what the U.S. Marines taught me . . . never give up and always accomplish the mission, no matter what. Never give up and keep focused on your perfect weight. You can and *will* do it.

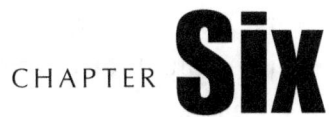

Summary

I HAVE ADDED this chapter to summarize the steps and re-quired daily action for this *Marine's Manual for Perfect Weight* to work. It will work and will *always* work if you accomplish the outlined steps that follow. Please reread this section every day, morning and evening.

1. Decide you want to get healthy and reach your perfect weight every day. The first day of the rest of your life is to-day, so read this each morning to get your mental attitude in a positive frame of mind. This is a mental program of seeing yourself as you want to be and deciding to make it happen. No one else can do this but you. Decide today to do some small exercise during the day and just do it. Decide today to eat a little healthier during the day and just do it.

2. Forgive yourself and anyone or anything who you current-ly blame for not being your perfect weight. When you or anyone says negative statements to you about weight, say the following to yourself: "I AM the captain of my own thoughts and the master of my body." Forgive yourself for setbacks but recognize you slipped up and start again now.

NOW is the first day of the rest of your life. Self-awareness is invaluable. Catch your negative thoughts and stop and replace them with positive thoughts. If you can do this every day, you will accomplish your mission of attaining and maintaining your own personal perfect weight. Why? Because you are now the captain of your thoughts, and what you think about all day long is what you become. I would say 95 percent of people never even watch what they are thinking about. Be one of the 5 percent who are in control of your weight and thoughts.

3. Imagine or visualize yourself at your perfect weight. See yourself in that swimming suit or wedding dress and believe you are there now. Have a conversation with a good friend or family member in your imagination about them telling you about how great you look and how super you feel. Your imagination is one of the keys to success in reaching and maintaining your perfect weight. Use your five senses (sight, sound, touch, smell, and taste) in your vision.

4. Repeat to yourself and memorize the following statement: "I AM so Happy and Grateful now that I AM a _____ pound healthy, loving, spiritual human being, and I AM getting better and better every day in every way." Repeat it to yourself constantly throughout the day. Say it when you are walking to your car, to the store, stuck in traffic, cooking, swimming, exercising . . . basically, during any of your day-to-day activities. When a negative thought pops up in your mind, see it and say to yourself, "get lost." Say, "I AM the captain of my thoughts and the master of my body." Remember, small wins every day make it impossible for you not to reach your goal. If you are positive more than 50 percent of the time, you are winning! Only you have control of your thoughts

and no one else. Never give up! Keep staying positive and watch your thoughts . . .

5. So as it is written, so let it be done. Write this statement down every day: "I AM so Happy and Grateful now that I AM a _____ pound healthy, loving, spiritual human being, and I AM getting better and better every day in every way" in your journal included in Chapter Seven. Then write the following: "I AM the captain of my thoughts and the master of my body."

6. The following are some helpful tips:

   a. Write your perfect weight statement, "I AM so Happy and Grateful now that I AM a _____ pound healthy, loving, spiritual human being, and I AM getting better and better every day in every way" on Post-it notes or index cards and post it all over your house, such as on your bathroom mirror, computer, TV, frig, by doorknobs; let your mind run wild . . .

   b. Post your perfect weight photo with your "I AM so Happy and Grateful now that I AM a _____ pound healthy, loving, spiritual human being, and I AM getting better and better every day in every way" statement on the back of your photos.

   c. Record your above mantra to your smartphone in your own voice and play it over and over with your earbuds on until you have completely memorized your mantra. Keep it up even when you do have it memorized for even better results.

   d. Look directly into your eyes reflecting in the mirror and repeat out loud to yourself the following: "I AM so Happy and Grateful now that I AM a _____ pound healthy, loving, spiritual being, and I AM getting better and better every day in every way." Remember the old saying that "your eyes are the gateway to your soul." Also, say to yourself while looking deep into your own eyes reflecting back from the mirror, "I love you, and I AM getting better and better every day in every way." You must love yourself and forget and forgive yourself and anyone else from the past.

e. Write me your success letter now. Put it in your journal. In 18 months, send it to me: Success@haspirits.com.

f. Do this program together with your husband or wife as a team. Best friends can team up and do this program as well. Mutual support never hurts.

g. Eat an apple each day to jog your thoughts to repeat your mantra. The old saying "An apple a day keeps the doctor way" is a good positive action to keep you focused on a positive attitude.

h. Join a gym or a training program when you decide you are ready. It will come to you naturally, like I said before, because *you* are the one deciding to reach your perfect weight, not some diet program.

i. Join a nutrition program when you decide to do it, not because someone told you to. Get my point; it is all on *you* to decide you want to become your perfect weight.

j. Create your own personal perfect weight mantra. It is OK to have as many as you want. The mantra must begin with I AM and be positive are the only requirements. The following are some examples:

1. I AM so happy and grateful now that I am a sexy, loving, 190 pound spiritual human being.

2. I AM so happy and grateful now that I AM a successful, loving 190 pound spiritual human being, and I AM getting better and better every day in every way.

3. I AM so happy and grateful now that I AM a lean 190 pound happy and healthy human being.

Journal

WRITE THE FOLLOWING in your own handwriting every day: "I AM so Happy and Grateful now that I AM a _____ pound healthy, loving, spiritual human being, and I AM getting better and better every day in every way." Also write the following: "I AM the captain of my own thoughts and the master of my body."

Additionally, write any positive win you had during the day. I have included some examples below regarding what I am talking about. It is your journal so just enjoy and have fun with it.

You have decided—now make it happen! Never give up and you will succeed. Period!

Example 1. I caught myself talking bad about someone and stopped midsentence. I told my bad thought to "get lost" and repeated my mantra, "I AM the captain of my own thoughts and the master of my body."

Example 2. I caught myself thinking negative thoughts over 20 times today and told those bad thoughts to "get lost." I AM the captain of my thoughts, and I repeated my personal mantra 10 times.

Example 3. I repeated my mantra, "I AM so Happy and Grateful now that I AM a _____ pound healthy, loving, spiritual human being, and I AM getting better and better every day in every way" over 200 times today, and I am beginning to understand that I am in charge of my life, and no one else.

Example 4. I walked around the block for the first time ever and said my mantra as I walked. I felt wonderful and in control of my life for the first time in a long time.

Example 5. I ate a salad today for lunch instead of the cheeseburger combo meal for the first time ever because I wanted to, not because someone told me to . . . I decided—no one else.

Example 6. I will never give up, and I now know that today is the first day of the rest of my life. Now I am in charge and driving my own bus to my perfect weight and health.

_____

_____

_____

_____

_____

_____

_____

_____

_____

WEEK_____

WEEK_____

WEEK_____

WEEK_____

WEEK_____

WEEK_____

WEEK_____

WEEK_____

WEEK_____

WEEK_____

WEEK_____

WEEK_____

WEEK_____

WEEK_____

WEEK_____

_____

_____

_____

_____

_____

_____

_____

_____

_____

_____

_____

_____

_____

WEEK_____

WEEK_____

WEEK_____

WEEK_____

WEEK

_____

_____

_____

_____

_____

_____

_____

_____

_____

_____

_____

_____

_____

_____

_____

_____

WEEK_____

_____

_____

_____

_____

_____

_____

_____

_____

_____

_____

_____

_____

_____

_____

_____

WEEK_____

WEEK _____

WEEK_____

WEEK_____

WEEK_____

WEEK_____

WEEK_____

WEEK_____

WEEK_____

WEEK_____

WEEK_____

WEEK_____

_____

_____

_____

_____

_____

_____

_____

_____

_____

_____

_____

_____

_____

WEEK_____

WEEK_____

WEEK_____

WEEK_____

WEEK_____

WEEK_____

WEEK_____

WEEK_____

WEEK_____

WEEK _____

WEEK_____

WEEK _____

WEEK_____

WEEK_____

WEEK_____

WEEK_____

WEEK _____

WEEK_____

WEEK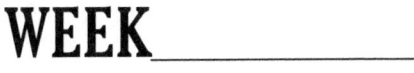

WEEK _____

WEEK_____

WEEK_____

WEEK_____

WEEK_____

_____

_____

_____

_____

_____

_____

_____

_____

_____

_____

_____

_____

_____

WEEK_____

WEEK_____

_____

_____

_____

_____

_____

_____

_____

_____

_____

_____

_____

_____

_____

_____

_____

WEEK_____

WEEK_____

WEEK_____

WEEK_____

WEEK＿＿＿＿＿

WEEK_____

WEEK_____

WEEK_____

WEEK_____

WEEK_____

WEEK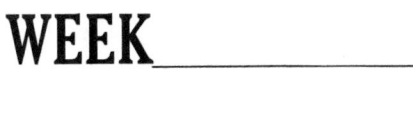

WEEK_____

WEEK_____

WEEK_____

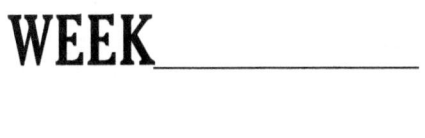

WEEK

WEEK_____